Table of Contents

Introduction

Welcome to "Functional Fitness: Efficient Workouts with Simple Equipment." In this guide, we'll explore the concept of functional fitness and how it can revolutionize your approach to exercise. Functional fitness focuses on building strength and mobility that directly translates to real-life activities, enabling you to move more efficiently and effectively in your everyday life. By incorporating functional movements into your workouts, you can improve your physical performance, prevent injuries, and enhance your overall quality of life.

The Essence of Functional Fitness

Functional fitness is all about training your body to handle real-life situations more effectively. Unlike traditional workouts that may isolate specific muscle groups, functional fitness emphasizes compound movements that engage multiple muscle groups simultaneously. This approach not only boosts your overall strength and flexibility but also enhances your coordination, balance, and endurance.

What to Expect in This Book

Throughout this book, we will dive deep into the principles of functional fitness and provide you with the knowledge and tools to implement it into your exercise routine. From understanding different exercise equipment to mastering bodyweight exercises and integrating functional movement patterns, we will cover all aspects of functional fitness.

Understanding Exercise Equipment

We will discuss the essential equipment needed for functional workouts, including resistance bands, kettlebells, and stability balls. You will learn how to select the right equipment based on your goals and available space. Each piece of equipment offers unique benefits and can be used in various ways to enhance your workouts.

Mastering Bodyweight Exercises

Bodyweight exercises are fundamental for building functional strength and mobility. Whether you are a beginner or an advanced exerciser, we will provide progressions and regressions for each exercise to ensure that everyone can benefit. You'll discover how to perform exercises like push-ups, squats, and lunges with perfect form and how to modify them to match your fitness level.

Maximizing Resistance Bands

Resistance bands are incredibly versatile and can be used for a wide range of exercises. We'll show you how to incorporate them into your routine to add resistance, enhance muscle activation, and improve overall strength. You'll learn exercises that target different muscle groups and how to adjust the tension to match your strength levels.

Exploring Kettlebell Training

Kettlebell training offers numerous benefits for functional fitness, such as improved strength, power, and coordination. We will introduce you to kettlebell exercises like swings, cleans, and snatches, and explain how they can enhance your functional fitness. You'll also learn how to safely incorporate kettlebells into your workouts and progress as you become more comfortable with the movements.

Integrating Functional Movement Patterns

Functional movement patterns are essential for improving mobility and preventing injuries. We will explore exercises that target specific muscle groups and enhance overall mobility. These exercises will help you move better and more efficiently in your daily life, from bending and lifting to twisting and reaching.

Core Strength and Stability

Core strength and stability are crucial for functional movement. We will provide you with exercises using simple equipment to develop a strong and stable core. A solid core is the foundation for all movements, and improving your core strength will benefit your overall fitness and help prevent injuries.

Cardiovascular Fitness in Functional Training

Cardiovascular fitness is not neglected in functional fitness. We will share strategies for improving your cardio health using simple equipment and creative exercises. You'll discover how to incorporate cardio into your functional training routines to enhance your endurance and overall fitness.

Creating Efficient Full-Body Workouts

Creating efficient full-body workouts is key to achieving your fitness goals. We will guide you on how to design workouts that target multiple muscle groups and movement patterns. You'll find sample workout routines and templates to maximize efficiency and effectiveness, ensuring you get the most out of your training sessions.

Progression, Recovery, and Long-Term Success

Finally, we will discuss the importance of progression, recovery, and long-term success. You will learn how to progress your functional fitness workouts, incorporate recovery strategies, and plan rest days to avoid burnout. Proper nutrition is also crucial, and we'll provide tips to support your long-term journey towards optimal health and fitness.

Ready to Begin?

Are you ready to embark on this transformative journey of functional fitness? Let's dive in and uncover the power of efficient workouts with simple equipment that will enhance your physical capabilities and improve your everyday life. Whether you're just starting out or looking to take your fitness to the next level, this book will be your guide to achieving and maintaining a healthier, more functional body. Let's get started!

Chapter 1: Understanding Functional Fitness

Functional fitness has become a buzzword in recent years, and for good reason. It focuses on exercises that mimic real-life activities and improve our overall strength and mobility. In this chapter, we will delve into the concept of functional fitness and its benefits for everyday life.

Introduction to the Concept of Functional Fitness

So, what exactly is functional fitness? Functional fitness involves performing exercises that replicate the natural movements we use in daily activities, such as bending, lifting, pushing, pulling, and twisting. Unlike traditional gym exercises that often isolate specific muscle groups, functional fitness emphasizes using multiple muscles and joints together. This approach enhances overall strength and mobility.

The beauty of functional fitness lies in its practicality. By training our bodies to move in ways that mirror everyday tasks, we can improve our balance, coordination, flexibility, and stability. Imagine how much easier carrying groceries, playing with children, or doing household chores would become. This type of fitness is about making life's daily demands more manageable and improving our overall quality of life.

Benefits of Functional Fitness for Everyday Life

Incorporating functional fitness into our routines offers numerous benefits. Let's explore some of the key advantages:

1. Improved Strength and Power: Functional movements engage multiple muscle groups simultaneously, leading to greater overall strength and power. This makes daily activities, such as lifting heavy objects or climbing stairs, much easier.

2. Increased Mobility and Flexibility: Functional fitness exercises involve dynamic movements that require a wide range of motion. Regular practice can improve joint mobility and flexibility, making it easier to perform tasks that require reaching, bending, and twisting.

3. Enhanced Balance and Coordination: As we age, our balance and coordination tend to decline. Functional fitness exercises challenge our proprioceptive abilities, improving our overall balance and coordination. This can help prevent falls and other injuries.

4. Injury Prevention: By training our bodies to move functionally, we develop strength in a balanced and coordinated manner. This can reduce the risk of injuries caused by muscle imbalances and improper movement patterns.

5. Increased Calorie Burn: Functional exercises often involve full-body movements, which require more energy and burn more calories compared to isolated exercises. This can contribute to weight loss and improved overall cardiovascular health.

Understanding the concept of functional fitness and its benefits helps us appreciate why it's essential to include functional movements in our fitness routines. Let's dive deeper into how this approach can transform our everyday lives.

Practical Application of Functional Fitness

Consider the daily activities we all engage in—whether it's bending down to pick something up, lifting a heavy bag, or simply walking up the stairs. Functional fitness aims to make these activities easier and more efficient. By practicing movements that mimic these tasks, we prepare our bodies to handle them with less effort and more ease.

For example, squats mimic the action of sitting down and standing up, lunges can improve the strength and balance needed for walking and running, and rotational exercises can enhance the twisting motions required for tasks like reaching for something on a high shelf.

Integrating Functional Fitness into Your Routine

Integrating functional fitness into your routine doesn't require fancy equipment or a gym membership. Many exercises can be performed using your body weight or simple household items. The key is to focus on movements that engage multiple muscle groups and mimic everyday actions.

Here are a few tips to get started:

- **Start with Basic Movements:** Begin with exercises like squats, lunges, push-ups, and planks. These foundational movements can be modified to match your fitness level and progressively made more challenging.
- **Use Household Items:** You don't need specialized equipment to perform functional exercises. Items like water bottles, chairs, and towels can be used for resistance and support.
- **Incorporate Variety:** To keep your routine interesting and effective, include a variety of movements that target different muscle groups and functional tasks.
- **Listen to Your Body:** Pay attention to how your body feels during and after workouts.

Ensure you maintain proper form to prevent injuries and maximize the benefits of your exercises.

Conclusion

Functional fitness is about preparing your body for real-life activities, enhancing your strength, mobility, balance, and coordination. By understanding and incorporating functional movements into your routine, you can improve your overall well-being and make everyday tasks easier and more enjoyable.

Now that we have a basic understanding of functional fitness, let's move on to Chapter 2, where we will explore the essential equipment needed for functional workouts. Get ready to take the next step in your functional fitness journey!

Chapter 2: Essential Equipment for Functional Fitness

In this chapter, we're going to delve into the essential equipment needed for functional workouts. The beauty of functional fitness is that it can be achieved with simple and affordable equipment that allows for a wide range of exercises. By incorporating these tools into your fitness routine, you can effectively target different muscle groups and improve overall strength and stability.

Overview of Equipment Options

When it comes to functional fitness, there are various equipment options that can enhance your workouts. Let's take a closer look at some key tools to consider:

1. **Resistance Bands:** Resistance bands are versatile and portable, making them an excellent choice for functional workouts. They provide varying levels of resistance and can be used for a wide range of exercises, such as squats, rows, and presses. Resistance bands are affordable and come in different strengths, allowing you to gradually increase the intensity as you progress.

2. **Kettlebells:** Kettlebells are compact and offer a unique training experience. They provide an excellent way to incorporate functional movements like swings, cleans, and snatches into your workouts. Kettlebells engage multiple muscles and joints, promoting functional strength, power, and coordination.

3. **Stability Balls:** Stability balls are great for improving balance, stability, and core strength. They can be used for various exercises, including planks, bridges, and stability ball crunches. Stability balls challenge your stability and require the activation of multiple muscle groups, enhancing your overall functional fitness.

Tips for Selecting the Right Equipment

When choosing equipment for your functional workouts, it's essential to consider your individual fitness goals and space constraints. Here are some tips to help you select the right equipment:

1. **Assess Your Goals:** Identify your specific fitness goals and determine which equipment will best help you achieve them. If your focus is on strength training, kettlebells and resistance bands may be ideal. If you're looking to improve balance and stability, stability balls could be the right choice.

2. **Consider Space:** Take into account the amount of space available for your workouts. If you have limited space, resistance bands and kettlebells are compact options that can be easily stored. Stability balls require more space but can still be a valuable addition to your routine if you have enough room.

3. **Start with the Basics:** If you're new to functional fitness, start with a few basic equipment pieces. Invest in a set of resistance bands with different resistance levels, as they provide a wide range of exercises and can be easily incorporated into any workout. As you become more comfortable, you can gradually add more equipment to diversify your routine.

4. **Seek Professional Advice:** If you're unsure about which equipment to choose or how to use it properly, consider consulting a fitness professional. They can provide guidance based on your individual needs and help you select the most suitable equipment for your goals.

Practical Advice for Using Equipment

Now that we've covered the types of equipment and tips for selecting the right tools, let's talk about how to use them effectively in your workouts:

- **Resistance Bands:** These are incredibly versatile. You can use them for resistance training, mobility exercises, and even stretching. For example, you can anchor a band under your feet for bicep curls or attach it to a door for rows.
- **Kettlebells:** When using kettlebells, focus on proper form to avoid injury. Start with basic movements like the kettlebell swing to build your strength and coordination. As you gain confidence, you can move on to more complex exercises like the Turkish get-up or snatch.
- **Stability Balls:** Stability balls can add an element of balance and core engagement to your workouts. Use them for exercises like ball squats, where you place the ball between your lower back and a wall, or for core exercises like stability ball rollouts.

Conclusion

By selecting the right equipment based on your goals and space constraints, you can create an effective functional fitness routine. In the following chapters, we will explore specific exercises and workouts using these essential tools, allowing you to maximize the benefits of functional fitness.

Remember, functional fitness is all about improving your ability to perform everyday activities with ease. With the right equipment and a well-rounded approach, you'll be well on your way to achieving greater strength, stability, and overall fitness.

Chapter 3: Mastering Bodyweight Exercises

Bodyweight exercises are a cornerstone of functional fitness. They require no equipment and can be performed anywhere, making them accessible to people of all fitness levels and abilities. In this chapter, we'll delve into mastering fundamental bodyweight exercises that will enhance your functional strength and mobility.

Understanding Bodyweight Exercises

Bodyweight exercises are movements that use the weight of your own body as resistance. They engage multiple muscles and joints, improving your overall strength, flexibility, and mobility. These exercises mimic everyday movements, making them highly functional and beneficial for real-life activities.

Benefits of Bodyweight Exercises

Incorporating bodyweight exercises into your fitness routine offers several key advantages:

1. **Convenience**: Bodyweight exercises can be performed anywhere, without the need for any equipment. Whether you're at home, in a park, or traveling, you can always fit in a workout.

2. **Accessibility**: Suitable for all fitness levels, bodyweight exercises can be modified to accommodate beginners and advanced individuals alike. By adjusting the intensity, range of motion, or adding variations, you can tailor the exercises to your specific needs and abilities.

3. **Functional Strength**: These exercises focus on movements that mimic daily activities, helping to improve your functional strength. This means you can perform everyday tasks, like carrying groceries or lifting objects, with ease and efficiency.

4. **Full-Body Engagement**: Bodyweight exercises engage multiple muscle groups and joints simultaneously, leading to a more efficient and effective workout. They promote better muscle balance, coordination, and stability.

Fundamental Bodyweight Exercises

To build a strong foundation in bodyweight training, let's explore a few fundamental exercises:

1. **Squats**: A basic lower body exercise that targets your quadriceps, hamstrings, and glutes. Stand with your feet hip-width apart, lower your hips back and down while keeping your chest lifted, then push through your heels to return to standing.

2. **Push-ups**: This exercise primarily targets your chest, shoulders, and triceps. Begin in a plank position with your hands slightly wider than shoulder-width apart, lower your chest towards the floor while keeping your core engaged, then press back up.
3. **Lunges**: Lunges work your quadriceps, hamstrings, and glutes. Start by standing with your feet hip-width apart, step forward with one leg, lower your body by bending both knees until your back knee is hovering above the ground, then push through your front heel to return to the starting position.
4. **Plank**: An excellent exercise for core strength and stability. Start in a push-up position, but instead of resting on your hands, place your forearms on the floor. Keep your body in a straight line from head to toe, engage your core, and hold for the desired duration.

Progressions and Regressions

To accommodate all fitness levels, bodyweight exercises can be progressed or regressed. Here are some tips:

- **Progressions**: Once you've mastered the basic form of a bodyweight exercise, make it more challenging by adding variations or increasing the range of motion. For example, elevate your feet during push-ups or perform pistol squats instead of regular squats.

- **Regressions**: If an exercise is too challenging, regressions can make it more manageable. You can decrease the range of motion, modify the exercise by using a stable support, adopt a kneeling position, or perform fewer repetitions.

Sample Bodyweight Workout

To get you started, here's a sample bodyweight workout routine that targets all major muscle groups:

1. **Bodyweight Squats**: 3 sets of 10-12 repetitions
2. **Push-ups**: 3 sets of 8-10 repetitions
3. **Reverse Lunges**: 3 sets of 10-12 repetitions per leg
4. **Plank Hold**: 3 sets of 30-45 seconds

Remember to warm up before starting the workout and cool down afterward. Listen to your body and adjust the intensity and repetitions according to your fitness level.

Conclusion

Mastering bodyweight exercises is a crucial step toward achieving functional strength and mobility. By incorporating these fundamental movements into your fitness routine and progressing at your own pace, you'll build a solid foundation for further functional fitness development. Start with the basics, focus on proper form and technique, and gradually challenge yourself to reach new levels of strength and mobility.

So, let's get started on mastering these bodyweight exercises. Your journey to enhanced functional fitness begins now!

Chapter 4: Maximizing Resistance Bands

Resistance bands are versatile and affordable tools that can greatly enhance your functional workouts. They offer a unique form of resistance that can target specific muscle groups, improve overall strength, and enhance stability. In this chapter, we'll dive into various techniques for incorporating resistance bands into your functional fitness routine, and explore creative exercises and workout routines that provide a full-body training experience.

Targeting Specific Muscle Groups

Resistance bands come in a variety of resistance levels, making them suitable for individuals of all fitness levels. Whether you're a beginner or an advanced athlete, resistance bands can be easily adjusted to match your strength and fitness goals. Here are some techniques for effectively targeting specific muscle groups using resistance bands:

Upper Body

1. **Bicep Curls:** Step on the band with one foot and hold the handles in each hand. Curl your arms up, focusing on contracting your biceps. This exercise helps in building bicep strength and tone.

2. **Lat Pulldowns:** Anchor the band overhead and hold the handles with your arms extended. Activate your lats and pull the band down towards your chest. This targets the latissimus dorsi muscles in your back.

3. **Push-Ups with Resistance:** Wrap the band around your back and hold the ends in your hands. As you perform push-ups, the resistance from the band will engage your chest, shoulders, and triceps even more, adding intensity to a classic exercise.

Lower Body

1. **Squats with Resistance:** Place the resistance band under your feet and hold the handles at shoulder height. As you squat down, the band provides added resistance, targeting your glutes, quads, and hamstrings. This enhances the effectiveness of the traditional squat.

2. **Glute Bridge:** Lie on your back with the band wrapped just above your knees. Push through your heels and lift your hips, engaging your glutes and hamstrings. This is great for building lower body strength and stability.

3. **Side Leg Lifts:** Anchor the band to a sturdy object and wrap it around your ankles. Lift one leg out to the side against the resistance of the band, targeting your outer

thigh muscles. This exercise helps in strengthening the hip abductors.

Full-Body Functional Training

In addition to targeting specific muscle groups, resistance bands can also be used for full-body functional training. By simulating real-life movements, these exercises engage multiple muscles and joints, promoting improved overall strength, stability, and mobility. Here are some creative exercises and workout routines that utilize resistance bands for full-body functional training:

1. **Band Pull-Aparts:** Hold the band with your hands shoulder-width apart, and keep your arms extended in front of you. Pull the band apart, squeezing your shoulder blades together and engaging your upper back muscles. This exercise improves posture and upper body stability.
2. **Standing Woodchoppers:** Anchor the resistance band at chest height. Stand perpendicular to the anchor point and hold the handles with both hands. Rotate your torso and pull the band diagonally across your body, simulating a woodchopping motion. This targets your core, obliques, and upper body muscles.
3. **Band-Assisted Pull-Ups:** Loop the resistance band around a secure overhead bar and step onto the band with your feet.

As you pull yourself up, the band provides assistance, making the pull-ups more achievable. This exercise strengthens your back, shoulders, and arms.

4. **Resistance Band Circuits:** Combine multiple resistance band exercises into a circuit training workout. Perform exercises such as squats, rows, lunges, push-ups, and shoulder presses using resistance bands. This high-intensity workout challenges your entire body and improves cardiovascular fitness.

Tips for Using Resistance Bands

1. **Start with the Right Resistance:** Choose a band with a resistance level that matches your current strength and fitness level. As you get stronger, you can progress to bands with higher resistance.
2. **Focus on Form:** Proper form is crucial to prevent injuries and maximize the effectiveness of your exercises. Ensure that you maintain good posture and controlled movements throughout each exercise.
3. **Gradually Increase Intensity:** As you become more comfortable with the exercises, gradually increase the intensity by using bands with higher resistance or by increasing the number of repetitions and sets.

4. **Mix It Up:** Keep your workouts interesting
    and challenging by incorporating a variety of
    exercises and changing your routine
    regularly. This prevents boredom and
    promotes continuous improvement.

Conclusion

Incorporating resistance bands into your functional
workouts can significantly enhance your strength,
stability, and mobility. They are an excellent
addition to any fitness routine, providing a versatile
and effective way to work out at home or on the go.
Experiment with different exercises and resistance
levels to find what works best for you. Remember
to maintain proper form and gradually increase the
intensity and resistance as you progress.

Now, let's move on to the next chapter to explore
the benefits of kettlebells in functional fitness.

Chapter 5: Unleashing the Power of Kettlebells

Introduction to Kettlebell Training

Kettlebell training has become immensely popular in recent years, and it's easy to see why. This chapter will introduce you to the world of kettlebell training and uncover its numerous benefits for functional fitness. Get ready to unleash the power of kettlebells and elevate your workouts to the next level.

Kettlebells are a unique piece of equipment that resemble a cannonball with a handle. They are known for their versatility and ability to provide both cardiovascular and strength benefits. Unlike traditional weightlifting, kettlebell training engages multiple muscle groups and promotes functional movements that mimic real-life activities.

One of the primary benefits of kettlebell training is improved overall strength. When performing exercises with kettlebells, you are not isolating specific muscles but rather engaging multiple muscle groups simultaneously. This leads to increased muscle activation and improved functional strength.

In addition to strength, kettlebell training enhances power—the ability to generate force quickly. The explosive movements involved in kettlebell exercises, such as swings and snatches, help develop power by improving the efficiency and coordination of your muscles. Coordination is another key area targeted by kettlebell training. Due to the dynamic nature of these exercises, you must coordinate your movements to smoothly transition between exercises and maintain proper form. This improved coordination carries over to your daily life, making everyday activities more fluid and efficient.

Kettlebell Exercises for Total-Body Strength

Kettlebell exercises are incredibly effective for developing total-body strength and functional movement patterns. Here are a few key exercises you can incorporate into your workouts:

1. Kettlebell Swing

The kettlebell swing targets your posterior chain muscles, including your glutes, hamstrings, and lower back.

How to do it:

- Stand with your feet shoulder-width apart and hold the kettlebell with both hands between your legs.

- Bend your knees slightly, hinge at the hips, and swing the kettlebell forward, maintaining a neutral spine.
- Drive through your hips to bring the kettlebell up to shoulder height, keeping your arms straight.
- Repeat the movement in a controlled manner.

2. Goblet Squat

The goblet squat is an excellent exercise for strengthening your lower body, particularly your quadriceps and glutes.

How to do it:

- Hold the kettlebell with both hands at chest height, close to your body.
- Stand with your feet slightly wider than shoulder-width apart and toes turned slightly outward.
- Lower your body by bending at the hips and knees, keeping your chest lifted and weight in your heels.
- Go as low as you comfortably can and then push through your heels to return to the starting position.

3. Kettlebell Clean and Press

This exercise targets your upper body, specifically your shoulders, arms, and core.

How to do it:

- Start with the kettlebell on the ground in front of you.
- Bend your knees and hinge at the hips to grab the kettlebell handle with one hand.
- Stand up explosively, using the momentum to bring the kettlebell up to your shoulder.
- From here, press the kettlebell overhead, fully extending your arm.
- Lower the kettlebell back to your shoulder and then down to the ground.
- Repeat on the other side.

Kettlebell Circuits for Functional Fitness

To enhance your functional fitness, kettlebell circuits are an excellent training method. Circuits involve performing a series of exercises back-to-back with minimal rest, providing a cardiovascular challenge while also targeting strength and coordination. Here is a sample kettlebell circuit you can try:

1. **Kettlebell Swing** - 10 repetitions
2. **Goblet Squat** - 10 repetitions
3. **Kettlebell Clean and Press** - 8 repetitions on each side

4. **Kettlebell Renegade Rows** - 8 repetitions on each side

Complete the circuit, resting for approximately 1 minute between rounds. Aim to complete 3-4 rounds, gradually increasing the weight and intensity as your fitness level improves.

Conclusion

Kettlebell training is a powerful tool for improving functional fitness. From increased strength and power to enhanced coordination, this versatile equipment can take your workouts to new heights. Incorporate kettlebell exercises and circuits into your routine to develop total-body strength and functional movement patterns.

Are you ready to unleash the power of kettlebells and achieve your fitness goals? Let's do it!

Chapter 6: Integrating Functional Movement Patterns

Functional movement patterns are fundamental movements that replicate real-life activities and are essential for everyday tasks and athletic performance. These movements improve mobility, strength, stability, and coordination, allowing you to move efficiently and without pain. By incorporating functional movement exercises into your workouts, you can enhance your overall fitness and improve your ability to perform daily activities with ease.

Understanding Functional Movement Patterns

Functional movement patterns involve multiple joints and muscles working together in a coordinated manner. They mimic movements we commonly perform in our daily lives, such as squatting, bending, twisting, pushing, pulling, and walking. By training these movement patterns, we can improve our ability to perform these tasks more effectively and with less risk of injury.

The importance of functional movement patterns lies in their ability to make our bodies move as a whole unit, rather than isolating individual muscles or joints. This integrated approach engages multiple muscle groups and joints simultaneously, enhancing overall stability, strength, and mobility.

Incorporating Functional Movement Exercises

Integrating functional movement exercises into your workouts can bring numerous benefits, not just for your everyday activities but also for your athletic performance. Here are some tips on how to effectively incorporate these exercises into your fitness routine:

1. Assess Your Movement Patterns:

Before diving into functional exercises, take the time to assess your current movement patterns. Identify any areas of weakness or limitations. This assessment will help you tailor your exercises to address specific areas that need improvement. You can do this yourself or with the help of a fitness professional.

2. Include a Variety of Movements:

Incorporate a variety of functional movement patterns into your workouts. This includes exercises that involve squatting, lunging, rotating, pushing, pulling, and balancing. By including a wide range of movements, you ensure that you are training your body to move in all planes of motion, which enhances overall functionality.

3. Use Functional Equipment:

Utilize functional equipment such as stability balls, resistance bands, and kettlebells to add variety and challenge to your workouts. These tools can help improve your balance, coordination, and stability. For example, kettlebell swings are great for building power and strength, while resistance bands can add an extra challenge to your squats and lunges.

4. Focus on Form and Technique:

Proper form and technique are crucial when performing functional movement exercises. This ensures that you are engaging the correct muscles and joints, reducing the risk of injury. If you're new to these exercises, consider working with a trainer to learn the correct form.

5. Progress Gradually:

Start with exercises that match your current fitness level and gradually progress as you become stronger and more comfortable with the movements. Progression can involve increasing resistance, adding complexity, or increasing the number of repetitions. For instance, you might start with bodyweight squats and eventually progress to weighted squats with a kettlebell.

6. Incorporate Balance and Core Stability Exercises:

Balance and core stability are key components of functional movement. Include exercises that challenge your balance and engage your core muscles, such as single-leg squats, plank variations, and stability ball exercises. These exercises will not only improve your functional strength but also help in preventing injuries.

Practical Examples of Functional Exercises

To give you a more concrete idea, here are some practical examples of functional exercises you can integrate into your routine:

- **Squats and Lunges:** These mimic movements like sitting down and standing up or stepping forward to pick something up.
- **Push-Ups and Pull-Ups:** These replicate the actions of pushing and pulling objects in daily life.
- **Planks and Stability Ball Exercises:** These enhance core strength and stability, which are essential for almost every movement.
- **Rotational Movements:** Exercises like Russian twists help improve the strength and mobility needed for tasks that involve twisting, like reaching for something on a shelf.

Conclusion

By incorporating functional movement exercises into your workouts, you can enhance your mobility, stability, and overall fitness. These exercises not only prepare you for daily activities but also improve your performance in sports or other physical pursuits. Remember to consult with a fitness professional to ensure that you are performing the movements correctly and to customize your workouts based on your individual needs and goals.

Good luck with your functional fitness journey, and enjoy the benefits of integrating functional movement patterns into your workouts. Embrace the process, and you'll soon find yourself moving with more ease and efficiency in every aspect of your life.

Chapter 7: Building Core Strength and Stability

Functional fitness isn't complete without focusing on core strength and stability. The core muscles play a crucial role in supporting functional movements and overall fitness. A strong and stable core improves posture, balance, and overall performance in daily activities and athletic endeavors. In this chapter, we'll dive into why core strength and stability are so essential and explore various exercises and workouts using simple equipment to enhance core strength.

The Importance of Core Strength and Stability

The core muscles, which include the abdominals, obliques, lower back, and hip muscles, serve as the center of the body's strength and stability. They act as a link between the upper and lower body, providing support for movements and transferring force efficiently. Having a strong and stable core is crucial for functional movement and overall fitness for several reasons:

Improved Functional Movement

Functional movements, such as bending, lifting, twisting, and reaching, heavily rely on core strength and stability. A strong core provides a sturdy foundation for these movements, allowing you to perform them with proper form and prevent injuries.

Better Posture

A weak core can lead to poor posture, which can result in muscle imbalances, back pain, and decreased mobility. By strengthening the core muscles, you can improve your posture, maintain a neutral spine, and alleviate any discomfort or pain caused by poor alignment.

Enhanced Balance and Stability

The core muscles play a significant role in balance and stability. By strengthening these muscles, you can improve your ability to maintain balance during functional movements, such as walking on uneven surfaces or reaching for objects in various positions. This increased stability also reduces the risk of falls and injuries.

Injury Prevention

A strong core provides stability and support to the spine, reducing the risk of lower back injuries. It also helps in transferring forces efficiently, minimizing the strain on other muscles and joints. Developing core strength and stability can prevent injuries during daily activities and sports participation.

Core-Focused Exercises and Workouts

Improving core strength and stability doesn't require complicated or expensive equipment. You can effectively target your core muscles using simple equipment and bodyweight exercises. Here are a variety of core-focused exercises and workouts that can help you improve your core strength, posture, balance, and stability:

Plank Variations

The plank exercise is a staple core exercise that targets the entire core musculature. Begin by assuming a push-up position with your elbows directly under your shoulders and forearms resting on the ground. Engage your core by pulling your belly button towards your spine and holding the position for a designated amount of time. As you progress, try different plank variations such as side plank, plank with leg lifts, or plank with shoulder taps to challenge your core from different angles.

Mountain Climbers

Mountain climbers are a dynamic exercise that targets not only the core but also the hip flexors and cardiovascular system. Start in a high plank position with your hands directly under your shoulders. Alternate driving your knees towards your chest while keeping your core engaged and your back flat. Increase the intensity by picking up the pace or performing mountain climbers on a stability ball or using resistance bands.

Russian Twists

Russian twists are an effective exercise for targeting the obliques, which are crucial for rotational movements and stability. Sit on the ground with your knees bent and feet flat on the floor. Lean back slightly while keeping your back straight and your core engaged. Holding a weight or medicine ball, twist your torso from side to side while maintaining a stable core. Increase the challenge by lifting your feet off the ground or using heavier weights.

Stability Ball Exercises

Stability balls are versatile tools that can add an extra element of instability to traditional core exercises, further engaging the core muscles. Exercises such as stability ball pikes, stability ball rollouts, and stability ball crunches target the core muscles while also challenging stability and balance.

Dead Bugs

Dead bugs are a fantastic exercise for core stability. Lie flat on your back with your arms extended towards the ceiling and your legs bent at a 90-degree angle. Slowly lower one arm and the opposite leg towards the ground while maintaining a stable core. Return to the starting position and repeat on the other side. Focus on keeping your lower back pressed into the floor and your core engaged throughout the movement.

Pilates and Yoga Movements

Both Pilates and yoga offer a wide range of movements and exercises that target the core muscles. Incorporating exercises like the Pilates Hundred, boat pose, or plank variations from a yoga class can help strengthen and stabilize your core.

Creating a Core-Focused Workout Routine

To maximize the benefits of core-focused exercises, it's important to incorporate them into a well-rounded workout routine. Here's an example of a core-focused workout routine using the exercises mentioned above:

- **Warm-up:** Perform 5-10 minutes of light cardio activity, such as jogging or jumping jacks.
- **Plank:** Hold a plank for 30 seconds, rest for 15 seconds, and repeat for a total of 3 sets.
- **Russian Twists:** Perform 3 sets of 12-15 repetitions, resting for 30 seconds between sets.

- **Stability Ball Rollouts:** Perform 3 sets of 10-12 repetitions, resting for 30 seconds between sets.
- **Dead Bugs:** Perform 3 sets of 10 repetitions per side, resting for 30 seconds between sets.
- **Mountain Climbers:** Perform 3 sets of 45 seconds, resting for 15 seconds between sets.
- **Cool-down:** Stretch the core muscles with exercises such as a seated forward fold or child's pose.

Remember to listen to your body and adjust the intensity and duration of the exercises based on your fitness level. As you progress, challenge yourself by increasing the weight, adding resistance bands, or incorporating more difficult variations of the exercises.

Conclusion

Building core strength and stability is crucial for functional movement and overall fitness. By incorporating core-focused exercises and workouts into your fitness routine, you can improve posture, balance, and core strength, ultimately enhancing your overall performance and reducing the risk of injury. So, don't neglect your core muscles—make them a priority in your functional fitness journey.

Chapter 8: Enhancing Cardiovascular Fitness

Cardiovascular fitness is a vital part of overall health and physical fitness. It refers to the ability of the cardiovascular system—which includes the heart, blood vessels, and lungs—to efficiently deliver oxygen and nutrients to the working muscles during exercise. In this chapter, we will explore strategies for improving cardiovascular fitness using functional cardio exercises and circuits. We'll also discuss creative ways to incorporate simple equipment for effective cardio workouts at home or in limited spaces.

Understanding Cardiovascular Fitness

Before diving into the strategies for enhancing cardiovascular fitness, it's essential to understand why this component of fitness is so important. Improving cardiovascular fitness offers a wide range of benefits, including:

- **Increased Endurance:** A stronger cardiovascular system allows you to sustain physical activity for longer periods without feeling fatigued.
- **Improved Heart Health:** Regular cardiovascular exercise strengthens the heart muscle, lowers blood pressure, and reduces the risk of heart disease.

- **Enhanced Calorie Burn:** Cardio exercises help burn calories, contributing to weight loss and weight maintenance.
- **Boosted Mood and Mental Health:** Engaging in cardiovascular workouts releases endorphins, which can improve mood, reduce stress, and alleviate symptoms of depression and anxiety.
- **Better Sleep:** Regular cardio exercise can enhance the quality of sleep, promoting better rest and recovery.

Functional Cardio Exercises

Functional cardio exercises are movements that engage multiple muscle groups and elevate the heart rate, thereby improving cardiovascular fitness. These exercises can be performed without any equipment, making them accessible for everyone. Here are a few examples of functional cardio exercises:

- **Jumping Jacks:** Stand with your feet together, then jump while spreading your legs wide and raising your arms overhead. Jump back to the starting position and repeat.
- **High Knees:** Stand tall and jog in place while lifting your knees as high as you can.
- **Burpees:** Start in a standing position, squat down, and kick your legs back into a push-up position. Perform a push-up, jump

your feet back to your hands, then explosively jump up, reaching your arms overhead.

- **Mountain Climbers:** Begin in a plank position, then alternate bringing one knee towards your chest while the other leg remains extended. Alternate quickly between legs, as if climbing a mountain.
- **Jump Rope:** Jumping rope is a classic cardio exercise that can be done virtually anywhere. If you don't have a jump rope, you can mimic the motion without it.

Functional Cardio Circuits

To maximize the benefits of cardiovascular exercise, you can create circuits that combine different functional cardio exercises. Circuits involve performing a series of exercises back-to-back with minimal rest in between. Here's an example of a functional cardio circuit:

1. **Jumping Jacks:** Perform 30 seconds of jumping jacks.
2. **High Knees:** Jog in place, lifting your knees as high as possible, for 30 seconds.
3. **Burpees:** Complete 10 reps of burpees.
4. **Mountain Climbers:** Perform 30 seconds of mountain climbers.
5. **Jump Rope:** Jump rope for 1 minute.
6. **Rest:** Take a 1-minute rest.

7. **Repeat:** Complete the circuit 3-4 times, resting for 1 minute between each circuit.

By incorporating circuits into your workouts, you can elevate your heart rate, challenge your cardiovascular system, and improve your overall fitness.

Using Simple Equipment for Effective Cardio Workouts

While functional cardio exercises can be done without any equipment, incorporating simple equipment can add variety and intensity to your workouts. Here are some creative ways to use common, inexpensive equipment for effective cardio workouts:

1. **Jump Rope:** As mentioned earlier, jumping rope is a fantastic cardio exercise. It can be done indoors or outdoors, making it a convenient option for limited spaces.
2. **Resistance Bands:** Attach a resistance band to a sturdy anchor point and perform exercises like standing rows or bicep curls. The resistance provided by the bands adds an extra challenge to your movements, requiring more effort from your cardiovascular system.
3. **Step-Ups:** Use a low platform or step and perform step-ups, alternating between your legs. This exercise elevates your heart rate

while also engaging your lower body muscles.

4. **Kettlebell Swings:** Hold a kettlebell with both hands and hinge at your hips to swing the kettlebell between your legs, then explosively drive your hips forward to swing the kettlebell up to shoulder height. This exercise not only improves cardiovascular fitness but also works your glutes, hamstrings, and lower back.

5. **Running or Cycling:** If you have access to a treadmill or stationary bike, you can incorporate running or cycling into your cardio routine to further challenge your cardiovascular fitness.

Remember to choose equipment that suits your fitness level and the available space. Start with equipment that you are comfortable with and gradually progress as you become more confident and experienced.

Conclusion

Improving cardiovascular fitness is integral to overall health and wellness. By incorporating functional cardio exercises and circuits into your fitness routine, you can enhance endurance, strengthen your heart, and reap the many benefits associated with cardiovascular exercise. Whether you choose to perform bodyweight exercises, use simple equipment, or a combination of both, the key is to engage in activities that elevate your heart rate and challenge your cardiovascular system. Stay consistent, listen to your body, and enjoy the journey towards improved cardiovascular fitness.

Next, in Chapter 9, we will discuss techniques for creating efficient full-body workouts that target multiple muscle groups and movement patterns.

Chapter 9: Creating Efficient Full-Body Workouts

When it comes to getting the most out of your fitness routine, designing efficient full-body workouts that target multiple muscle groups and movement patterns is key. In this chapter, we'll explore techniques for creating these workouts, provide sample routines, and offer templates to help you maximize efficiency and effectiveness in your fitness journey.

Designing Efficient Full-Body Workouts

The goal of functional fitness is to engage multiple muscle groups and movement patterns in a single workout. This approach not only saves time but also ensures you're getting the most comprehensive workout possible. Here are some techniques to help you design efficient full-body workouts:

1. **Compound Movements**: Incorporate exercises that involve multiple joints and muscle groups. Examples include squats, deadlifts, push-ups, and rows. These exercises allow you to work multiple muscles simultaneously, making your workout more efficient.
2. **Supersets and Circuits**: Perform exercises back-to-back with minimal rest between

sets. This technique keeps your heart rate elevated and maximizes calorie burn. You can create supersets by pairing exercises that target different muscle groups, such as squats followed by push-ups. Alternatively, you can design circuits that involve a series of exercises performed one after another.

3. **Incorporate Plyometrics**: Plyometric exercises, also known as jump training, are explosive movements that help increase power and improve cardiovascular fitness. Examples include box jumps, jump squats, and burpees. Adding plyometrics to your workout routine can further enhance the efficiency of your full-body workouts.

4. **Use Functional Equipment**: Incorporate functional equipment like resistance bands, kettlebells, and stability balls into your workouts. These tools can add variety and intensity to your exercises, targeting different muscle groups and movement patterns. For example, you can integrate resistance bands into your squats or use kettlebells for swings and presses.

Sample Workout Routines and Templates

To help you get started, here are two sample workout routines that emphasize efficiency and full-body engagement:

Sample Workout Routine 1: Full-Body Superset

1. **Squats** - 3 sets of 10 reps - Rest 30 seconds
2. **Push-Ups** - 3 sets of 10 reps - Rest 30 seconds
3. **Bent-over Rows** - 3 sets of 10 reps - Rest 30 seconds
4. **Lunges** - 3 sets of 10 reps per leg - Rest 30 seconds
5. **Shoulder Press** - 3 sets of 10 reps - Rest 30 seconds
6. **Plank** - 3 sets of 30 seconds - Rest 30 seconds

Sample Workout Routine 2: Full-Body Circuit

Perform each exercise for 45 seconds, then rest for 15 seconds before moving on to the next exercise. Complete 3 rounds.

1. **Kettlebell Swings**
2. **Resistance Band Rows**
3. **Stability Ball Hamstring Curls**
4. **Push-Ups**
5. **Romanian Deadlifts**
6. **Mountain Climbers**
7. **Russian Twists**
8. **Jumping Lunges**

Feel free to customize these sample routines based on your fitness level, goals, and available equipment. You can also mix and match exercises to create your own unique full-body workouts.

Customizing Your Workouts

When customizing your workouts, consider the following:

1. **Fitness Level**: Adjust the number of sets, repetitions, and rest periods according to your fitness level. Beginners might start with fewer sets and longer rest periods, while more advanced individuals can increase the intensity and reduce rest times.
2. **Goals**: Tailor your workouts to align with your specific fitness goals. If you're aiming to build strength, focus on exercises that allow you to lift heavier weights. If your goal is to improve cardiovascular fitness, incorporate more high-intensity interval training (HIIT) and plyometric exercises.
3. **Equipment Availability**: Make use of the equipment you have. If you don't have access to certain tools, modify the exercises accordingly. For instance, if you don't have kettlebells, use dumbbells for swings or presses.

Tips for Maximizing Efficiency

1. **Warm-Up and Cool Down**: Always start with a warm-up to prepare your muscles and joints for the workout ahead. Likewise, end with a cool down to help your body recover.
2. **Proper Form and Technique**: Focus on maintaining proper form and technique to prevent injuries and maximize the effectiveness of your exercises.
3. **Progression**: Gradually increase the intensity of your workouts over time to continue challenging your body and promoting growth.
4. **Consistency**: Stick to a regular workout schedule to see the best results. Consistency is key to achieving long-term fitness goals.

By targeting multiple muscle groups and movement patterns in a single session, you can save time and maximize the effectiveness of your training. Remember, the most efficient workouts are those that keep you engaged, challenge your body, and align with your fitness goals. So, start designing your efficient full-body workouts today and enjoy the benefits of a more comprehensive and effective fitness routine!

Chapter 10: Progression, Recovery, and Long-Term Success

As you embark on your functional fitness journey, it's crucial to understand how to keep challenging your body and achieving new fitness goals. Progression involves gradually increasing the intensity, duration, or difficulty of your exercises to elicit further improvements in strength, endurance, and mobility. In this chapter, we'll discuss how to effectively progress your workouts, the importance of recovery, and strategies for ensuring long-term success.

Guidance on Progressing Functional Fitness Workouts

To continue challenging your body and achieving new fitness goals, it is essential to have a plan for progressing your functional fitness workouts over time. Here are some guidelines to help you progress effectively:

1. Set Specific and Realistic Goals:

Before starting any fitness program, it is important to set specific and realistic goals. Determine what you want to achieve with your functional fitness training. Whether it's increasing your strength, improving your mobility, or enhancing your overall fitness, having clear objectives will help you design an effective progression plan. For example, you might aim to lift a certain weight, run a specific distance, or achieve a new level of flexibility.

2. Gradually Increase Intensity:

As you become more comfortable and proficient with your workouts, it's important to gradually increase the intensity. This can be achieved by adding resistance, increasing the number of repetitions or sets, or shortening rest periods. Avoid making sudden jumps in intensity as this can lead to overexertion or injuries. Instead, aim for small increments in intensity over time to allow your body to adapt and progress safely. For instance, if you're lifting weights, consider increasing the load by a small percentage every few weeks.

3. Experiment with Different Exercises and Variations:

To continue challenging your body and prevent plateaus, try incorporating new exercises and variations into your routine. Experiment with different movement patterns that target the same muscle groups but in slightly different ways. This variation not only keeps your workouts engaging but also helps to recruit different muscles and improve overall functional strength. For example, if you regularly do standard push-ups, try adding in some decline push-ups or push-ups with a twist.

4. Utilize Different Training Methods:

In addition to varying the exercises, incorporate different training methods into your workouts. This could include interval training, circuit training, or high-intensity interval training (HIIT). By constantly challenging your body with different training approaches, you can maximize your progress and prevent boredom. Each method brings unique benefits: interval training improves cardiovascular fitness, circuit training builds endurance and strength, and HIIT boosts metabolism and burns calories.

Importance of Recovery Strategies, Rest Days, and Proper Nutrition

While pushing your body during workouts is important for progress, it is equally important to prioritize recovery and rest. Without adequate recovery, your body can become overworked and susceptible to injuries. Here are some strategies to help with recovery and promote long-term success:

1. Allow Sufficient Rest Days:

Rest days are crucial for adequate recovery. They allow your muscles, joints, and nervous system to recover from the stress of exercise. Aim for at least one or two rest days per week, during which you engage in low-intensity activities or take complete rest. Listen to your body and adjust the frequency and intensity of your workouts accordingly. Rest days are not a sign of weakness; they are an essential part of your training plan.

2. Incorporate Active Recovery:

Active recovery refers to engaging in low-intensity activities or exercises that promote blood flow and help facilitate recovery. This could include light stretching, foam rolling, or engaging in low-impact activities such as yoga or swimming. Active recovery can help reduce muscle soreness, improve flexibility, and enhance overall recovery. For example, a gentle yoga session can help relax your muscles and mind after a week of intense workouts.

3. Prioritize Proper Nutrition:

Proper nutrition plays a vital role in supporting your long-term functional fitness success. Fueling your body with balanced meals that include an adequate amount of protein, carbohydrates, and healthy fats helps support muscle repair and growth. Additionally, staying hydrated is crucial for optimal performance and recovery. Consider consulting a nutritionist to create a meal plan that aligns with your fitness goals.

4. Listen to Your Body:

It's important to listen to your body and pay attention to any signs of fatigue or injury. Pushing through pain or discomfort can lead to overtraining and setbacks. If you experience persistent pain or feel excessively fatigued, take a break or consult with a healthcare professional. Being mindful of your body's signals helps prevent long-term injuries and ensures sustainable progress.

5. Get Adequate Sleep:

Sleep is a critical component of recovery. Aim for seven to nine hours of quality sleep each night to allow your body to repair and recharge. Sleep deprivation can negatively impact your performance, recovery, and overall well-being. Establish a regular sleep schedule and create a relaxing bedtime routine to improve your sleep quality.

Conclusion

By incorporating progression strategies, prioritizing recovery, and maintaining a healthy lifestyle, you can set yourself up for long-term success in your functional fitness journey. Remember, progress takes time, and consistency is key. Stay committed, stay patient, and enjoy the rewards of functional fitness in your everyday life. As you continue to challenge yourself and adapt your workouts, you'll find that the benefits extend far beyond physical improvements, enhancing your overall quality of life.